Diabetes

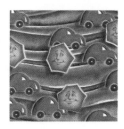

what you should know

b

**Blackwell
Science**

Diabetes

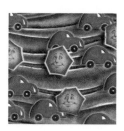

what you should know

Written by Dean J. Kereiakes, MD, FACC,
and Douglas Wetherill, MS
Illustrated by Laura L. Seeley

©2001 by Robertson & Fisher Publishing Company. Second Edition.

Written by: Dean J. Kereiakes, MD, FACC; and Douglas Wetherill, MS
Contributing Editors: Paul Ribisl, PhD; Rona Wharton, MEd, RD, LD; Charles J. Glueck, MD, PhD;
                       and Dirk Iwema
Illustrated by: Laura L. Seeley

Distributors:
Blackwell Publishing
c/o AIDC
P.O. Box 20, 50 Winter Sport Lane, Williston, VT 05495-0020 USA
(Telephone orders: 800-216-2522; fax orders: 802-864-7626)

Blackwell Science, Ltd.
c/o Marston Book Services, Ltd.
P.O. Box 269, Abingdon, Oxon OX14 4YN, England
(Telephone orders: 44-01235-465500; fax orders: 44-01235-465555)

Printed in Canada
01 02 03 04 5 4 3 2 1 (ISBN:0-632-04531-0)

The Blackwell Science logo is a trademark of Blackwell Science Ltd., registered at the United Kingdom
Trade Marks Registry.

A catalog record for this book is available from the U.S. Library of Congress.

The authors would like to acknowledge the generous support of the following individuals for their support in the second edition: Angela Ginty and Paul Neff.

We would also like to extend our appreciation to The McGraw-Hill Companies for permission to use their adapted illustrations.

Treatment Disclaimer

This book is for education purposes, not for use in the treatment of medical conditions. It is based on skilled medical opinion as of the date of publication. However, medical science advances and changes rapidly. Furthermore, diagnosis and treatment are often complex and involve more than one disease process or medical issue to determine proper care. If you believe you may have a medical condition described in the book, consult your doctor.

Table of Contents

Introduction

Diabetes is a chronic disease that, left untreated, can be life-threatening. Yet nearly one-third of those who have diabetes are undiagnosed — and untreated. The American Diabetes Association estimates that, of the 15.7 million people in the United States who have diabetes, 5.4 million are undiagnosed, leaving them at great risk for serious complications.

What exactly is diabetes? Most people know that diabetes is related to sugar in the body. How does the body use sugar? Read on.

About Diabetes

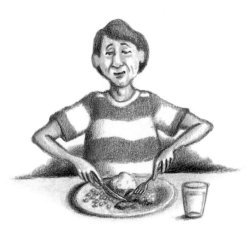

For our friend
Hartley,
mealtime
is called
"happy time."

2

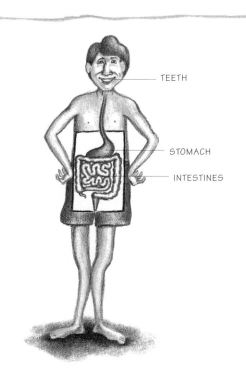

TEETH

STOMACH

INTESTINES

While Hartley eats, his digestive system (teeth, stomach, and intestines) breaks the food down into smaller particles that are used by his body.

3

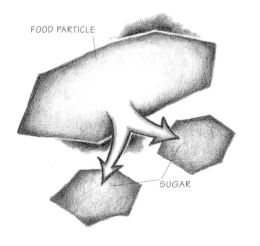

FOOD PARTICLE

SUGAR

Some food is broken down into particles of **sugar**. Sometimes this sugar is referred to as **carbohydrates** or **glucose**.

Sugar moves from the digestive system to the blood and travels throughout the body to feed the working cells. The sugar is the energy packet the cells need to do work like running and breathing.

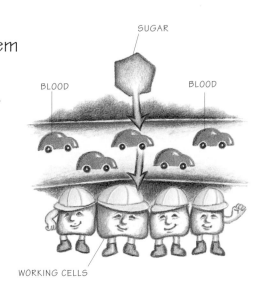

SUGAR

BLOOD

BLOOD

WORKING CELLS

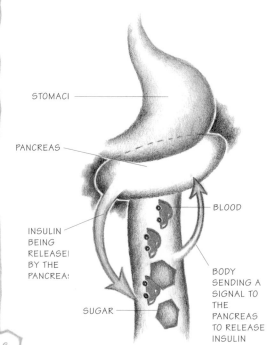

STOMACH

PANCREAS

INSULIN BEING RELEASED BY THE PANCREAS

SUGAR

BLOOD

BODY SENDING A SIGNAL TO THE PANCREAS TO RELEASE INSULIN

At the same time, the body sends a signal to the **pancreas** telling it to release **insulin** into the bloodstream. Insulin is released from the "beta" cells of the pancreas.

6

Insulin acts like a **key** that unlocks the doors of the cells to let sugar move in. The working cells can then use the sugar for energy to do their jobs. This is how your body uses sugar. However ...

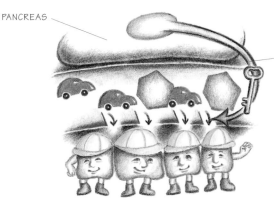

PANCREAS

INSULIN BEING RELEASED BY THE PANCREAS TO ALLOW SUGAR TO MOVE INTO THE WORKING CELLS

7

Without the key (insulin), the sugar cannot get out of the bloodstream and into the working cells. The sugar builds up in the blood, and the working cells get hungry. This is what happens in diabetes. A diabetic's body cannot move sugar from the blood into the cells.

Types of Diabetes

Type 1

Type 2

There are 2 reasons diabetics cannot move sugar from the blood to the cells.

One reason is that the body cannot produce insulin. This is known as **type 1** diabetes. A type 1 diabetic must take insulin injections to replace the missing insulin.

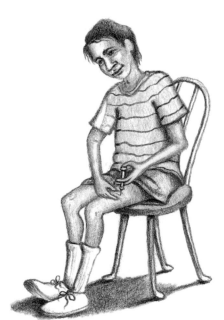

Remember, insulin is used by your body to feed your cells. Insulin must be injected every day. There are many places the shots can be given.

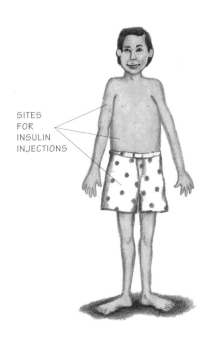

SITES FOR INSULIN INJECTIONS

The other type of diabetes is called **type 2**. This type of diabetes is a result of the body's resistance to insulin. Even if the body produces extra insulin, the sugar has a hard time getting from the blood to the working cells. Because of the extra work producing more insulin, the pancreas may wear out.

Type 2 diabetes affects 90% of all diabetics while ...

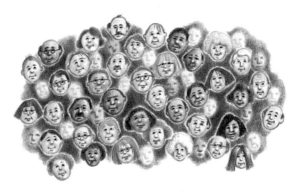

10% have type 1 diabetes.

Let's recap everything so far:

1) A **type 1 diabetic** cannot produce enough insulin.

2) A **type 2 diabetic** has insulin resistance with hyperinsulinemia (cannot use insulin effectively), does not produce enough insulin, or both.

Either type of diabetes may be dangerous to your health.

Both types of diabetes may result in **big trouble** if the diabetes is not controlled. If you have diabetes, you should keep your blood sugar level between 80 mg/dL and 130 mg/dL or other limits determined by your doctor. Only by testing your blood sugar **frequently** can you manage to control it between these limits.

The body works best when the blood sugar is within these limits. It is a constant struggle to walk the fine line between blood sugar that is too low and that which is too high.

Another, longer-term measure of blood sugar is called **glycohemoglobin**. The upper limit for glycohemoglobin should be 7%. (This test is discussed in more detail on pages 34-38. Read on!)

Too low

Low blood sugar can make you feel jittery, sweaty, and dizzy. If your blood sugar falls to very low levels (usually below 60 mg/dL), then you might even pass out.

This can be due to too much insulin, too much exercise, not enough carbohydrates, or excessive alcohol intake. It is very important that you eat some carbohydrates to boost your blood sugar back up to normal.

Too high

High blood sugars for long periods can cause damage to important body parts such as your eyes, kidneys, heart, skin, and nerves. In the short term, high blood sugar can cause excessive urination, excessive thirst, changes in vision, and increased likelihood of having bacterial or fungal infections.

High blood sugars may be due to not enough insulin, eating too much, some medications, or another illness which can interfere with glucose metabolism and can cause your blood sugar to go up.

19

If your blood sugar is too high, your body may start breaking down fat for fuel and start producing **ketones**.

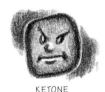

KETONE

Ketones

When the body does not receive energy from sugar, fats start breaking down to produce energy. If too many fats break down, they may be converted into a poison called **ketones**. Symptoms of too many ketones may include nausea, vomiting, increased heart rate and rapid breathing. Ultimately, a person producing ketones may end up in a coma.

A person with type 2 diabetes may not experience the same problems as someone with type 1 diabetes. However, it is important to know the dangers of diabetes and to work at keeping it under control.

Do You Have Any Symptoms?

What are the major signs you may have diabetes?

Generally, they are considered to be:

A) Frequent urination
B) Excessive thirst
C) Excessive hunger
D) Unexplained weight loss
E) Urinary tract infections
F) Red, itchy rash in the folds of the skin, usually caused by fungus

Other common symptoms that may occur separately or together include:

A) Fatigue
B) Blurred vision
C) Poor healing of cuts and scrapes
D) Dry mouth
E) Excessive or unusual infections
F) Impotence (in males)

OR

G) Lack of feeling or a "tingly" or burning
sensation in the hands or feet

These (G) are symptoms of neuropathy that
indicate the diabetes is affecting the peripheral
nerves.

**If you have any of these symptoms, you should
schedule an appointment with your doctor.**

What to Expect at Your Doctor's Office

How do you determine if you have diabetes?

Only your doctor can diagnose diabetes.

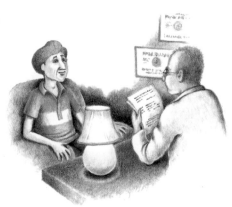

The test is very simple:

A) Do not eat or drink anything (except water) after midnight.
B) Go to your doctor the next morning to have your blood drawn after 8:00 a.m.
C) The sugar in your blood will be measured. Your doctor will be able to determine your **fasting blood sugar**.

The doctor may measure fasting serum insulin to better understand type 2 diabetes. If the insulin level is higher than 20 uU/ml, then you have hyperinsulinemia, caused by the cells in the body being resistant to the action of insulin.

A very important number to remember!

20

uU/ml

Just as important ...

If your **fasting blood sugar** is between 110 mg/dL and 125 mg/dL, the American Diabetes Association (ADA) says that you have **impaired glucose tolerance** or IGT.

Other important numbers to remember:

110 to 125

mg/dL

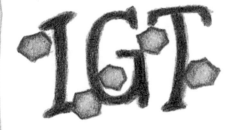

Why is impaired glucose tolerance or IGT important? Because if a person is at risk, he or she has a greater chance of eventually developing diabetes.

Type 2 diabetes can progressively worsen over time. However, it may be reversed if it is caught early. Someone who has a normal sugar response may gradually become inactive, overeat, and become overweight. He or she may develop insulin resistance and ultimately may increase the chances of developing diabetes.

It is important both you and your doctor develop a realistic and aggressive approach for dealing with diabetes.

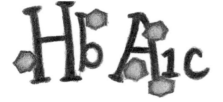

Your doctor may also ask you to have a hemoglobin A1c (Hb A1c) test to determine how controlled (close to normal) your blood sugar has been over the last 3 months.

How does this test work?

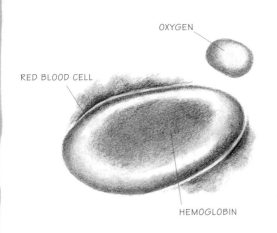

OXYGEN

RED BLOOD CELL

HEMOGLOBIN

This gets a little complicated. Hang in there.

Hemoglobin is a part of your blood.

35

When hemoglobin is around blood sugar, the sugar starts sticking to the hemoglobin.

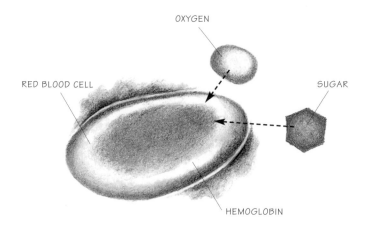

OXYGEN

RED BLOOD CELL

SUGAR

HEMOGLOBIN

The more sugar in the blood, the more it sticks to the blood cells. They become "sugar coated."

RED BLOOD CELL USED TO CARRY OXYGEN AND NUTRIENTS

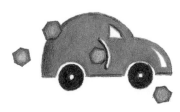

"SUGAR COATED" RED BLOOD CELL

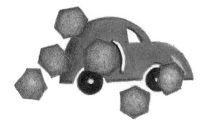

What are the normal values for Hb A1c?

Nondiabetic	Less than 6%
Diabetic in good control	Less than 7%
Diabetic out of control	Greater than 8%

Talk to your doctor about what your Hb A1c target should be.

According to the ADA, individuals should be tested for diabetes according to the following guidelines:

1) Testing should be done at age 45 and above. If the results are within normal limits, the individual should be rechecked every 3 years.
2) Testing should be considered before age 45 or should be carried out more often for people who:
   - Are overweight
   - Have a first-degree relative (parent, brother, or sister) with diabetes

- Are members of an ethnic population that is at high risk of developing diabetes (e.g., African-American, Hispanic, Native American)
- Have delivered a baby weighing more than 9 pounds, or have been diagnosed with **gestational diabetes mellitus**
- Have blood pressure above 140/90 mm Hg
- Have an HDL-cholesterol level less than 35 mg/dL and/or a triglyceride level more than 250 mg/dL
- Have been diagnosed with **impaired glucose tolerance** on a previous test

How Serious is Diabetes?

Complications of diabetes may include damage to the eyes, the kidneys, and the nerves (with "pins and needles" or painful feelings in the hands or feet). Diabetes also increases the risk of heart attack and stroke.

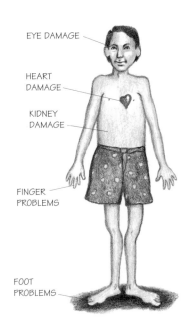

EYE DAMAGE

HEART DAMAGE

KIDNEY DAMAGE

FINGER PROBLEMS

FOOT PROBLEMS

The heart

The ADA reports that increased blood sugar levels may damage the heart 4 to 7 years before the symptoms of diabetes appear. In other words, damage may be occurring to the body, but the individual does not realize it. Diabetics are 2 to 4 times more likely to develop heart disease than nondiabetics. Consequently, they are more at risk of developing plaque in their arteries. If plaque clogs the arteries of the heart, blood flow to the heart muscle is reduced, and the heart muscle may not receive enough oxygen.

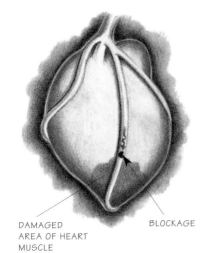

DAMAGED
AREA OF HEART
MUSCLE

BLOCKAGE

Lack of oxygen to the heart may cause a portion of the heart to be damaged. For more information on what contributes to plaque development, please see Appendix A, page 66.

Kidneys

The kidneys filter waste products out of the blood. If sugar-induced damage occurs to the kidneys, the kidneys may not be able to filter properly. This may cause **protein** to leak into the urine, which is a sign that something is wrong with the kidneys.

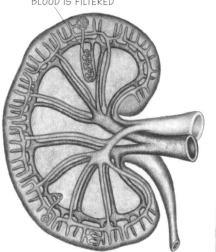

SMALL ARTERIES WHERE BLOOD IS FILTERED

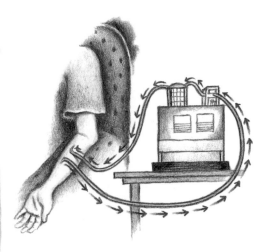

Dialysis

Poor kidney function is a common form of advanced disease for diabetics. If the kidneys start to fail, **dialysis** may be needed to remove waste from the blood.

Feet and fingers

Sugar can attach to the nerves and arteries that supply the fingers and feet. The damage to the nerves may result in one or more of the following symptoms:

1) Tingly, "pins and needles" feelings in the hands or feet
2) Burning pain in the hands or feet
3) Loss of feeling in the hands or feet (much less likely)

Damage to the arteries may limit blood flow to these areas.

Lack of proper attention to the lower legs and poor circulation are the leading causes of amputation for diabetics.

Eyes

Similarly, diabetics may have restricted blood flow to the eyes. The body may try to compensate by developing new arteries. These new arteries can cause scarring or can leak. The seeping blood may distort the retina, impair vision, and even cause blindness.

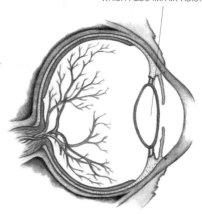

SUGAR MAY BUILD UP IN THE LENS OF THE EYE AND RESULT IN CATARACTS, WHICH ALSO IMPAIR VISION.

PERMISSION GRANTED BY THE McGRAW-HILL COMPANIES FOR USE OF ADAPTED ILLUSTRATION BY H. McMURTRIE AND J. RIKEL, *THE COLORING REVIEW GUIDE TO HUMAN ANATOMY*, 1991, Wm. C. BROWN PUBLISHERS.

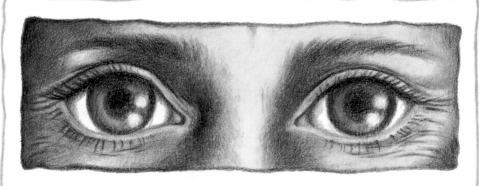

If you have had diabetes more than 5 years, or if you are 30 years old or older, it is important that you receive a yearly **eye exam. Ophthalmologists** use eye drops to dilate the pupils so that they can examine the blood vessels in the back of the eyes properly.

Treatment of Diabetes

Large research studies have reported that careful control of blood glucose may reduce complications. How can you achieve good control? Try these:

A) Self-monitoring of blood glucose
B) Diet
C) Staying as close as you can to ideal body weight
D) Education
E) Exercise
F) Medications
G) Attitude

Frequent self-monitoring of blood sugar

How often should you measure your blood sugar?

You should measure before each meal and before bedtime. Blood sugar may be measured at home, school, or work. This means diabetics should ideally monitor their blood sugar **4 times a day**.

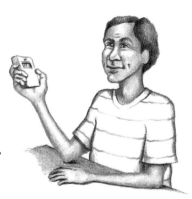

It is important to know what your blood sugar level is so you can take the correct action to adjust it. If your blood sugar level is **too low**, you may want to skip the next dose of oral medications for your diabetes or reduce the amount of insulin you take. You may also want to eat some sugar or hard candy, or drink some orange juice. If your sugar is **too high**, you may need a shot of insulin and, in rare instances, fluid or electrolyte replacement. People with type 2 diabetes may not need to test as often as those with type 1.

You should also test when you suspect that your blood sugar is not in control. Talk with your doctor about how often you should monitor your blood sugar. **You should always talk to your doctor before adjusting your oral medication or insulin.**

Diet

Because diabetes is about sugar, and sugar comes from what you eat, your diet becomes VERY important. You may have to meet with a **registered dietitian** to set up a meal plan just for you. And it will be a healthy way of eating!

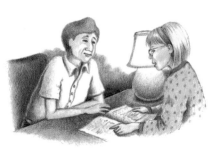

Unfortunately, one diet does not work for everyone with diabetes. The dietitian will generally review your lab results and lifestyle and then discuss treatment options. The diet becomes a form of treatment — **medical nutrition therapy** — which is just for you.

Education

Education is a major factor in controlling your diabetes. A **certified diabetes educator** can review how you monitor your blood sugar, provide you with the latest recommendations, and possibly suggest lifestyle changes.

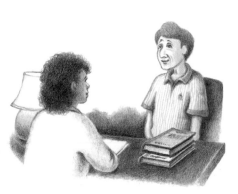

Exercise

Physical inactivity is related to the development of type 2 diabetes. So, exercise is very important. Exercise is also important to type 1 diabetics, but your food and insulin regimens may have to be changed to provide enough energy for exercise.

Because everyone is different, you should obtain approval from your doctor before you begin a vigorous exercise routine. Your diabetes educator or dietitian can help you with any changes.

Medications

As mentioned earlier, medication may
significantly improve your control of diabetes.
The 2 main types of medication include:

  1) Insulin (type 1)
  2) Oral medication (type 2)

1. Insulin

Type 1 diabetics cannot produce **insulin** and, therefore, need insulin injections. There are many types of insulin to help control blood sugar:

A) Insulin which is extracted from animals

B) Synthetic human insulin

Because various amounts of insulin are needed throughout the day, there are different types of insulin available. You and your doctor can work together to get the right insulin treatment for you.

2. Oral medication

Type 2 diabetes may be controlled by proper diet and exercise. If type 2 diabetes cannot be controlled by diet and exercise, you may need an oral medication or could require insulin.

There are 2 basic types of oral medicine for diabetes which work very differently:

A) Drugs which reduce insulin resistance and lower insulin levels by making the cells in the body more receptive to insulin. These drugs are called insulin "sensitizing" drugs. A recent study of one class of these drugs, biguanides, has shown the drugs to be very effective in reducing the complications of diabetes.

B) Another class of antidiabetic drugs (sulfonylureas) stimulates the pancreas to provide more insulin.

You should talk to your doctor about determining which class of medications is most effective for you.

Attitude

Diabetes is a serious disease. However, with an accepting attitude, you can live a normal, healthy life.

Start by being honest with yourself. You have to **want** to get in control. It requires a lot of discipline. If you are successful, there is less chance that diabetes will prevent you from doing what you want to do. And, ultimately, you can put diabetes in its proper perspective — allowing yourself to be a person first, and a diabetic second.

Appendixes

A. Risk factors for complications
B. Heart medications
C. Exercise
D. Questions

A. Risk factors for complications

After you have been diagnosed with diabetes, what risk factors may "complicate" your diabetes?

1) A family history of heart disease
2) Obesity
3) Cigarette addiction
4) High blood pressure above 130/85 mm Hg
5) Elevated total cholesterol above 200 mg/dL
   Elevated LDL-cholesterol above 100 mg/dL
   Low HDL-cholesterol below 40 mg/dL
   Elevated triglycerides above 250 mg/dL

1. Family history

A **family history** of cardiovascular disease could reflect genetics and/or an unhealthy family lifestyle. If most of your family members smoke, are sedentary, and have a poor diet — then these are harmful habits that increase the risk of heart disease in your family. However, unlike your genes, these behaviors can be changed.

On the other hand, if your family has a healthful lifestyle but there is still a high incidence of cardiovascular disease, then it is likely that genetics is playing a role. We are learning more about the importance of genetic risk for vascular disease. In the future, treatment may be tailored to an individual's own genetic makeup. In either case, by practicing a healthful lifestyle, you can help reduce your risk rather than giving up and thinking you have no control over your destiny.

2. Obesity

The American Heart Association has described obesity as a major risk factor for cardiovascular disease. What exactly is obesity?

Metropolitan Life's height/weight tables are often used to determine a recommended weight for an individual based on age and gender. Generally, those who are 20% over the recommended weight for their height are considered to be overweight — but not necessarily obese. Obesity refers to fatness rather than weight. Men who have greater than 25% of their body weight as fat and women who have more than 35% are considered to be obese. Obesity and being overweight carry significant health risks, are directly related to cardiovascular risk factors, and may:

1) raise triglycerides (a "bad" blood fat)
2) lower HDL-cholesterol (the "good" cholesterol)
3) raise LDL-cholesterol (the "bad" cholesterol)
4) raise blood pressure and
5) increase the risk of developing diabetes

Obesity may be related to both genetics (nature) and lifestyle (nurture). Generally speaking, obesity occurs when the calories we consume exceed the calories we burn through activities of daily living and exercise. We store the excess calories as fat reserves, thus contributing to obesity and ultimately increasing the risk of coronary disease. Obesity has increased in men and women in every decade over the past 50 years. There is a misconception that Americans are overeating and eating too much fat. In fact, as a nation we are eating less fat, fewer calories, and still gaining weight — primarily due to the lower levels of physical activity in our youth and adult lives. A sedentary lifestyle could be the real culprit.

3. What about smoking?

Don't do it. Smoking is bad for the entire cardiovascular system because it:

A) Introduces carbon monoxide into the body

B) Lowers the "good" HDL-cholesterol

Carbon monoxide

Oxygen attaches to the red blood cells in the lungs. Red blood cells transport the oxygen throughout the body.

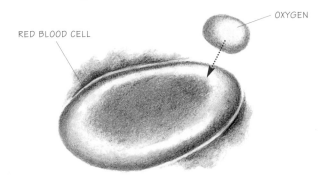

OXYGEN

RED BLOOD CELL

When you smoke, you inhale carbon monoxide into your lungs. Carbon monoxide binds to the red blood cells at the site where oxygen normally binds.

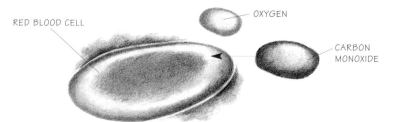

RED BLOOD CELL

OXYGEN

CARBON MONOXIDE

Therefore, less oxygen is carried by the blood, resulting in less oxygen available for use in the heart, muscles, and throughout the body. People who smoke may have abnormal heartbeats as well.

Understandably, smoking has harmful effects, especially for anyone who has already had a heart attack or bypass surgery. More importantly, there is an increased likelihood of a second heart attack or need for another bypass surgery if you continue to smoke after an initial cardiac incident.

Smoking is also a risk factor for peripheral vascular disease (blockages of the arteries to the brain, kidneys and legs).

Lower HDL-cholesterol

Two other reasons for
not smoking are that
it reduces the amount
of HDL-cholesterol or
"good cholesterol" in your
bloodstream, and it makes
your blood clot more easily,
increasing the potential
for an arterial blockage
(heart attack or stroke).

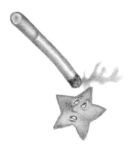

SMOKING
REDUCES
HDL-CHOLESTEROL

4. Hypertension

SYSTOLIC
NUMBER

140
_____
90

DIASTOLIC
NUMBER

Hypertension is commonly referred to as high blood pressure. If you have a **systolic pressure** greater than 140 mm Hg and/or a **diastolic pressure** greater than 90 mm Hg on 2 separate visits to the doctor, then you may have high blood pressure.

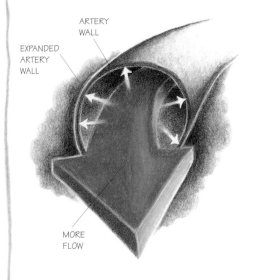

SYSTOLE

EXPANDED
ARTERY
WALL

ARTERY
WALL

MORE
FLOW

What is **systolic pressure**? Blood comes out of the heart in 1 big thrust. The artery expands to handle the blood. The amount of pressure put on the expanded artery wall is called **systolic pressure**.

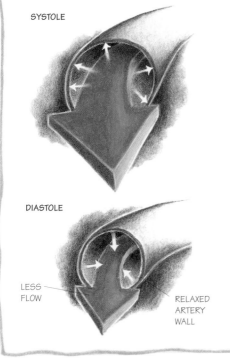

SYSTOLE

DIASTOLE

LESS FLOW

RELAXED ARTERY WALL

After the artery expands during systole, it relaxes back to its normal size. It is similar to a rubber band that goes back to its normal shape after being stretched. Normal pressure on the artery wall during relaxation is called **diastolic pressure**.

How does hypertension relate to cardiovascular disease?

Blood pressure is a result of the blood flowing through the artery (cardiac output) and the resistance of the artery wall (vascular resistance). If that sounds too technical, here ... this may help:

Blood pressure = Cardiac output x vascular resistance

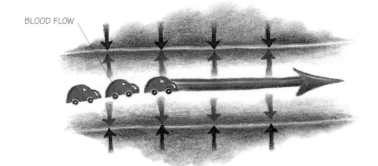

BLOOD FLOW

If a lot of resistance is created by either the blood or the artery wall, then there is more pressure as the blood travels through the artery. If it takes more energy to get the blood through the arteries, then your heart has to work harder with each beat. Most people with high blood pressure do not realize they have it. No wonder hypertension is called the "silent killer."

What contributes to hypertension?

Several factors may contribute to hypertension and cardiovascular disease. These include:

Excess dietary salt
Excess alcohol intake
Stress
Age
Genetics and family history
Obesity
Physical inactivity
High saturated fat diet

Salt

Salt helps conserve water in your body. The American Heart Association Step II Diet recommends that the average person consume no more than 2,400 mg of salt per day, especially those individuals who are salt sensitive. Excess dietary salt may contribute to both hypertension and to your body retaining too much water.

If you are retaining too much water, then you are increasing your blood volume (cars) without adding space. This increase will result in more pressure in the arteries.

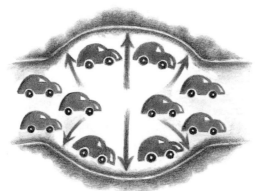

Alcohol consumption

A common concern for individuals with cardiovascular disease is alcohol consumption — mainly because there seems to be conflicting evidence about the benefits versus the risks of drinking. Experts agree that excess alcohol consumption over time can lead to many harmful effects, including high blood pressure, cirrhosis of the liver, and damage to the heart. The issue is the balance between **moderate** and **excessive** alcohol consumption. While the evidence shows that there is a protective effect for moderate alcohol consumption, this benefit disappears with excessive intake. Men should consume no more than 2 drinks* daily, and women, because of their smaller body size, should not consume more than 1 drink* each day. The 7 to 14 allowable drinks in a week should not be consumed in a few days or during a weekend of binge drinking. People who should not drink include individuals with high levels of triglycerides in their blood (over 300 mg/dL), women who are pregnant, individuals who are under age, people with a genetic predisposition for alcoholism or who are recovering from alcoholism, and those taking certain medications.

*A guide: One drink is defined as 5 ounces of wine, 12 ounces of beer, or 1-1/2 ounces of 80-proof liquor.

What about stress?

When you are under stress, your brain releases signals to the body through the nerves. These signals allow your body to respond to various situations.

Arteries have nerves attached to them. The nerves can either cause the arteries to relax or can put more tension on the walls of the arteries. If you are under a lot of stress, the nerves send signals to tighten or narrow the arteries.

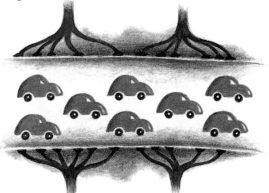

Narrowing the artery is like taking away a lane of traffic. There is still the same number of cars (blood) with less space (artery). This increases the pressure inside the artery.

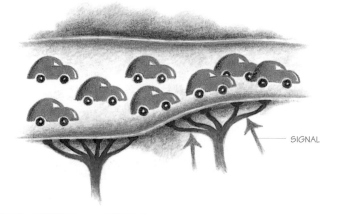

SIGNAL

So,

something you can do to improve your blood pressure is reduce stress. You can accomplish this by practicing meditation, doing deep breathing exercises, or doing exercise, such as going for a walk, riding a bike, or taking a swim.

5. Elevated cholesterol

Cholesterol is a "waxlike substance" that serves as a "building block" within the **cell membrane**.

CELL MEMBRANE

CHOLESTEROL

T
TESTOSTERONE

BILE ACID

E
ESTROGEN

Cholesterol is also used to make **hormones,** especially those found in reproduction: **estrogen** and **testosterone.**

Cholesterol is used to make **bile acids** that help break down fat in our intestines.

Why is cholesterol so harmful?

Fatty streaks in the arteries start to develop in the first decade of life as a result of **lipids** moving into the cell wall of the artery. These fatty streaks may become more advanced **atherosclerotic lesions** and may then progress to "advanced lesions" often referred to as **plaque**.

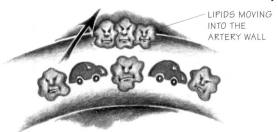

LIPIDS MOVING INTO THE ARTERY WALL

Plaque restricts the flow of blood through the artery, similar to orange construction barrels you have seen on the highway. Plaque reduces the flow of blood (traffic) and increases pressure in the artery (construction zone).

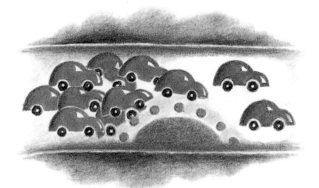

What should my cholesterol levels be?

For those individuals with coronary heart disease or diabetes, **LDL-cholesterol** should be **less than 100 mg/dL**. For individuals with two or more risk factors for cardiovascular disease, **LDL-cholesterol** should be **less than 130 mg/dL**.

Triglycerides should be **less than 200 mg/dL**.

HDL-cholesterol should be **greater than 40 mg/dL** for men and **more than 45 mg/dL** for women.

B. Heart medications

1. ACE (angiotensin converting enzyme) inhibitors, AII (angiotensin receptor) blockers and vasodilators

Say that 3 times fast! A major concern for diabetics is high blood pressure. It is recommended that the maximum resting blood pressure for diabetics be 130/85 mm Hg. These drugs act to enlarge the diameter of the arteries (reduce vascular resistance), thereby permitting an easier flow of blood and decreasing the workload of the heart. ACE inhibitors have been shown to reduce overall blood pressure in diabetics and also to protect the kidneys. ACE inhibitors are very important when a test of urine shows even a very small amount of protein caused by diabetes. This is called **microalbuminemia**.

These drugs may vary with respect to their peak effective daily dose and the required frequency of administration.

2. Aspirin

The ADA recommends
that aspirin be taken
by "high-risk" men and
women who have either
type 1 or type 2
diabetes and who are
at risk of developing
cardiovascular disease.

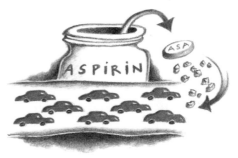

Ask your doctor if you would benefit from taking an enteric-coated aspirin. These aspirin usually come in doses of 81 mg or 325 mg. You may not be a candidate for aspirin therapy if you are allergic to aspirin, have a bleeding tendency, are already on anticoagulant therapy, or experienced recent gastrointestinal bleeding and/or liver problems.

Talk with your doctor before taking any medications, including aspirin.

C. Exercise

Before you start your exercise routine, there are a couple of things that you should do.

1) Monitor your blood glucose

2) Check your feet

Glucose too high

Before and after any exercise session, you should monitor your blood glucose. If your blood sugar is too high (more than 240 mg/dL), you must test your urine for ketones. This requires a special test strip. If ketones are present in your urine, you should not exercise. Call your doctor.

Glucose too high before exercise

240

mg/dL

Test for ketones in urine.

Glucose too low

If your blood sugar is too low (less than 100 mg/dL), you probably do not have enough energy to carry out the entire exercise session. You should eat a light snack with 15 grams of carbohydrates — such as a piece of fruit or a couple of graham crackers.

Glucose too low before exercise

100

mg/dL

Eat a light snack with 15 grams of carbohydrates.

Glucose just right

If your blood sugar is **just right** — between
100 mg/dL and 240 mg/dL — we'll just call you
Goldilocks. Go ahead and exercise!

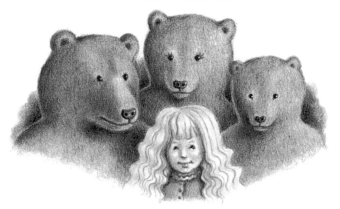

Shoes

For diabetics,
important pieces of
exercise equipment
are the proper shoes
and socks for walking
or jogging.

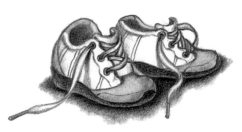

Select shoes that fit your feet properly. Shoes that are either too tight or too loose may cause your feet to develop blisters or sores. These areas may become infected.

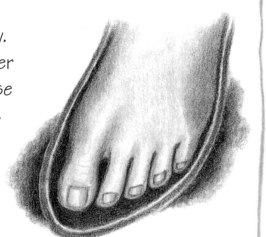

Sock selection is equally important. During exercise, even your feet perspire. Select polypropeline socks which will transmit sweat away from your foot to the shoe and to the atmosphere. This will help prevent your feet from chafing.

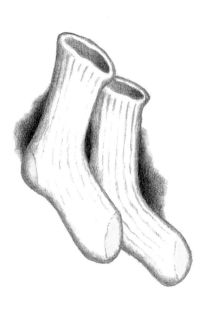

Be sure that you:

A) Clean your feet thoroughly with soap and warm water after you exercise.

B) Completely dry your feet.

C) Check your feet for any open sores or blisters.

D) Put on fresh socks.

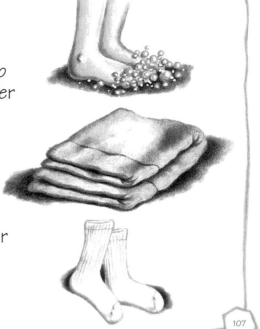

Currently, only 22% of adults in the United States exercise at a level that benefits their cardiovascular systems. What are some important considerations?

1) Type of exercise

2) Amount and regularity of exercise

3) Intensity of exercise

You should always consult with your doctor about type and duration of exercise prior to beginning an exercise routine.

1. Type of exercise

To meet your general fitness goals, the best type of exercise is **aerobic** exercise. Aerobic exercise does not necessarily require special equipment or a health club membership. Aerobic exercises are those that require a lot of oxygen. These exercises include walking, jogging, cycling, swimming, cross-country skiing, or rowing.

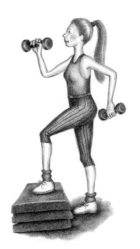

20-30 minutes a day, 5 days a week

2. Amount and regularity of exercise

The U.S. surgeon general recommends that healthy adults exercise 20 to 30 minutes, 5 days a week.

There are nearly 50 half hours in a 24-hour day. Exercising for 30 minutes daily requires **only about 2%** of your total day. Try to find 1, or 2, or 3 exercises you like to do. You'll enjoy the variety.

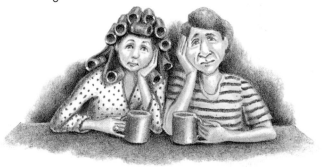

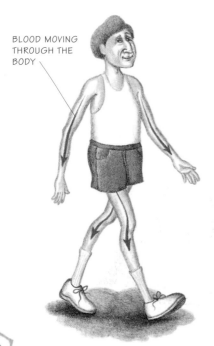

BLOOD MOVING
THROUGH THE
BODY

3. Intensity of exercise

Warm up

By walking or cycling
slowly, you move the
blood out to the
working muscles.
A warm-up should
start slowly and
last 5 to 10 minutes.

You cannot maintain "all out" exercise (100%) for very long. An example of an "all out" exercise is sprinting. Actually, you may only maintain a sprint for about 15 seconds.

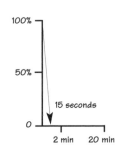

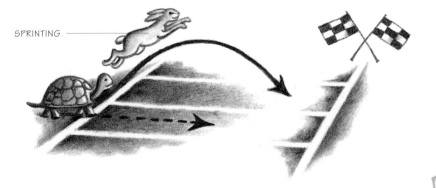

SPRINTING

113

If you slow the exercise down a bit, to about 90%, you may still only go for about 2 minutes!

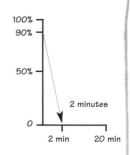

100%
90%

50%

2 minutes

0

2 min   20 min

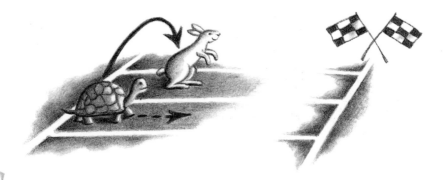

What if you slow your exercise down to 75% or even 50%? There is a **huge** difference. Now, you may easily go more than 20 minutes.

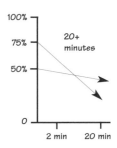

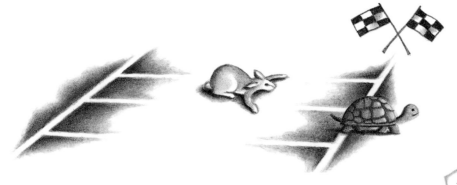

Simply —

By slowing down the pace, you may be able to exercise for a longer period of time.

Many exercise physiologists use the following generally accepted formula to determine the exercise target heart rate of a healthy individual. If you have a history of cardiovascular disease, or if you are just starting a program, **check with your doctor before starting an exercise routine**. Your doctor is aware of the many factors that may need to be considered in modifying your exercise intensity.

Target heart rate example

Your age: 50

1. 220 minus your age:
2. Answer #1 minus
   your resting pulse:
3. Answer #2 x 0.5:
4. Answer #3 plus
   your resting pulse:
5. Answer #2 x 0.75:
6. Answer #5 plus
   your resting pulse:
7. **Target heart rate** equals
   range between values for
   #4 and #6:

Your resting pulse: 70

1. 220 - 50 = 170

2. 170 - 70 = 100
3. 100 x 0.5 = 50

4. 50 + 70 = 120
5. 100 x 0.75 = 75

6. 75 + 70 = 145
7. **120 to 145 beats
   per minute, or 12 to 14
   beats for 6 seconds**

Now it's your turn

Here is how you determine the heart rate of an apparently healthy individual. Please consult with your doctor to make sure that this is an accurate target heart rate for your condition.

1. Measure your pulse (heart rate) for 60 seconds: _____
2. Take 220 and subtract your age: 220 - _____ = _____
3. Now take the answer in #2 and subtract your pulse: _____
4. Take the answer in #3 and multiply by 0.5: _____
5. Take the answer in #4 and add your pulse: _____
6. Take the answer in #3 and multiply by 0.75: _____
7. Take the answer in #6 and add your pulse: _____
8. Your target heart rate should range from the answer in #5 (_____) to the answer in #7 (_____).
9. Divide each answer in #8 by 10 to determine your pulse for 6 seconds: _____ to _____ .

How hard and how often should I exercise?

When you are just starting out, try to exercise very comfortably. Here are 4 quick tips.

1) Try to exercise so that you are breathing noticeably but are **not** out of breath. Remember this simple rule: you should be able to carry on a conversation while you are exercising.

2) Sweating is a good thing. This means that your body is working hard enough and receiving the necessary stimulus for the muscles and the heart.

3) If you are not fatigued and are completely recovered from exercising on the previous day, then you should exercise **daily**.

4) Give yourself a **warm-up** before exercise (several minutes of easy walking) and a **cooldown** at the end of exercise (again, several minutes of easy walking). Ask an exercise specialist for some recommendations for stretching after your workout, and discuss the intensity of the exercise with your doctor.

Important!

To begin your exercise program, it may be advantageous for you to exercise only 15 to 20 minutes daily for the first few weeks. This may help you more easily establish a consistent exercise routine. Check with your doctor for input on your exercise program.

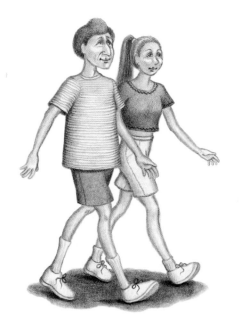

If you are just starting an exercise program, probably the simplest exercise to try is walking. It is fairly easy to do for 20 minutes.

123

VERY, VERY important

Cool down. As important as the warm-up and the aerobic exercise are to improving your fitness, you must also include a cooldown as part of your exercise routine.

Your cooldown should be just like your warm-up. At the end of your exercise routine, give yourself 5 to 10 minutes of nice, easy walking. You also may want to include some mild stretching.

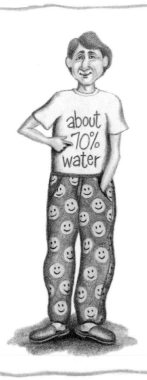

Another consideration – water

Water is needed for virtually every function of the body. The body is approximately 70% water.

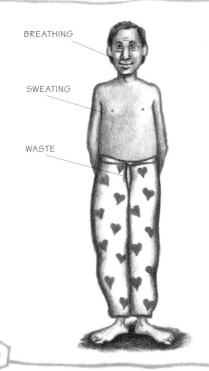

BREATHING

SWEATING

WASTE

During the course of the day, you lose water through sweating, breathing, and waste. Replacement of water (rehydration) is important — especially when participating in an exercise program.

A prudent recommendation is that you should drink 6 to 10 glasses of water per day. Sorry, caffeinated drinks and alcohol do not count. They are "diuretics," meaning that they actually may cause you to lose even more water.

D. Questions

Here are some questions that you may want to take with you the next time you go to see your doctor.

What are my medications? How does each of them help me?

Answer _____

_____

_____

_____

_____

_____

_____

Should I have a treadmill test before I start to exercise? What is my target heart rate?

Answer _____

_____

Do I have any *exercise limitations* of which I should be aware?

Answer _____

_____

Based on my blood glucose levels, blood pressure, and blood cholesterol levels, should I talk to someone about changing my diet?

Yes   No

Contact your local hospital for the name of a registered dietitian.

Dietitian _____

Address _____

_____

Phone _____

Whew! That is a lot of information packed into a tiny book. The reality is that diabetes is very complicated. You simply cannot take one tablet a day and forget about it. Diabetes requires constant attention. However, large research studies have reported that diabetics who strive to lower their Hb A1c to less than 7% greatly reduce the number of complications associated with diabetes.

So, where should you start? Well, first talk to your doctor. His or her goal is to help you help yourself.

Your doctor can direct you to invaluable resources, including a certified diabetes educator and a registered dietitian. Then, if your doctor approves, you should get started on a simple exercise program — mainly walking. You may not be able to completely reverse your condition, but you can take simple steps that may lead to a more complete and healthier life.

Bibliography

American College of Sports Medicine Position Stand, "The Recommended Quality and Quantity of Exercise for Developing and Maintaining Cardiorespiratory and Muscular Fitness in Healthy Adults." *Medicine and Science Sports and Exercise* April 1990.

American Heart Association Consensus Panel Statement. "Preventing Heart Attack and Death in Patients With Coronary Disease." *Circulation* 1995; 2-4.

Burke, A.P., and A. Farb, G.T. Malcom, Y. Liang, J. Smialek, R. Virmani, "Coronary Risk Factors and Plaque Morphology in Men with Coronary Disease Who Died Suddenly." *New England Journal of Medicine* 1 May 1997: 1276-1282.

Collins, R., and R. Peto, C. Baigent, P. Sleight. "Aspirin, Heparin, and Fibrinolytic Therapy in Suspected Acute Myocardial Infarction." *New England Journal of Medicine* 20 March 1997: 847-860.

Da Costa, F.D., et al. "Myocardial Revascularization with the Radial Artery: A Clinical and Angiographic Study." *Annals of Thoracic Surgery* Aug. 1996: 475-480.

The Diabetes Control and Complications Trial Research Group. The effect of intensive treatment of diabetes on the development and progression of long-term complications in insulin-dependent diabetes mellitus. *New England Journal of Medicine* 1993, 329: 977-986.

Eckel, R.H. "Obesity in Heart Disease," *Circulation* 1997: 3248-3250.

Executive Summary of the Third Report of the National Cholesterol Education Program (NCEP) Expert Panel on Detection, Evaluation, and Treatment of High Blood Cholesterol in Adults (Adult Treatment Panel III). JAMA, May 16, 2001, Vol. 285, No. 19: 2486-2497.

Freidman, G.D., and A.L. Klatsky. "Is Alcohol Good for Your Health?" *New England Journal of Medicine* 16 Dec. 1993: 1882-1883.

Glueck, C.J., and J.E. Lang. "Lipoprotein metabolism in the elderly." *The Merck Manual of Geriatrics.* Abrams, W.B., M.H. Beers, R.B. Berkow, eds. Merck and Co. Rahway, N.J. 1995: 1023-1025.

Grossman, E., and F.H. Messerli. "Diabetic and Hypertensive Heart Disease." *Annals of Internal Medicine.* 51996; 125: 304-310.

Kannel, W.B., R.B. D'Agostino, and J.L. Cobb. "Effects of Weight on Cardiovascular Disease" Am J Clin Nutr 1996; 63 (suppl): 419S-422S.

Kenney, W.L. et al. *American College of Sports Medicine Guidelines for Exercise Testing and Prescription,* 5th ed. Media, Pa.: Williams & Wilkins, 1995.

Margolis, S., and P.J. Goldschmidt-Clermont. The Johns-Hopkins White Papers. Baltimore: The Johns-Hopkins Medical Institutions; 1996: 1-66.

McCarron, D.A., and M.E. Reusser. "Body Weight and Blood Pressure Regulation" Am J Clin Nutr 1996; 63 (suppl): 423S-425S.

Meeker, M.H., and J.C. Rothrock. Alexander's Care of the Patient in Surgery, 10th Ed. St. Louis: Mosby; 1995: 1058-1122.

Peterson, J.A., and C.X. Bryant. *The Fitness Handbook;* 2nd Ed. St. Louis: Wellness Bookshelf; 1995.

Schlant, R.C., and R.W. Alexander. The Heart, 8th Ed. New York: McGraw-Hill, 1994: 892-1102.

Superko, H.R. "The Most Common Cause of Coronary Heart Disease can be Successfully Treated by the Least Expensive Therapy — Exercise." *Certified News* 1998: 1-5.

United States Surgeon General on his priorities at http://www.osophs.dhhs.gov/myjob/priorities.htm accessed November 1999.

Voors, A.A., et al. "Smoking and Cardiac Events After Venous Coronary Bypass Surgery." *Circulation.* Jan. 1, 1995, Vol. 93, No. 1: 42-47.

Zelasko, C.J. "Exercise for weight loss: What are the facts?" J Am Diet Assoc 1995; 95: 973-1031.

About the Authors

Dean J. Kereiakes, MD, FACC, is one of the nation's preeminent cardiologists. Dr. Kereiakes is President of the Ohio Heart Health Center, Medical Director of the Carl and Edyth Lindner Center for Clinical Cardiovascular Research, Professor of Clinical Medicine at the University of Cincinnati, and Professor of Medicine at The Ohio State University. He frequently lectures worldwide and has published hundreds of articles and papers. Dr. Kereiakes lives in Cincinnati, Ohio.

Douglas Wetherill, MS, is Supervisor of Disease Management at a large Midwest manufacturing company. He lives in Cincinnati, Ohio.

For additional copies of *Diabetes: What You Should Know™,*
please contact your local bookseller or call (800) 216-2522

For institutional quantities, contact our Special Sales Department at
rsime@blacksci.com or call (800) 759-6102

Other titles in the series *Your Health: What You Should Know™:*

Congestive Heart Failure: What You Should Know™
Heart Disease: What You Should Know™
High Cholesterol: What You Should Know™
Women's Health Over 40: What You Should Know™
Women's Health Under 40: What You Should Know™